Your Amazing
Itty Bitty®

Guide for Adult
20/20 Vision Loss

*15 Key Topics for Successful Lifestyle
Modifications*

Gloria Riley

Published by Itty Bitty® Publishing
A subsidiary of S & P Productions, Inc.

Printed in the United States of America

Itty Bitty Publishing
311 Main Street, Suite D
El Segundo, CA 90245
(310) 640-8885

ISBN: 978-1-950326-13-6

This information is for educational purposes only and is not intended as a substitute for medical advice, diagnosis, or treatment. You should not use this information to diagnose, or to treat a health problem or eye condition yourself.

This guidebook is dedicated to everyone, especially "Baby Boomers", who are struggling with vision loss. It's intended to raise public awareness and offer a better understanding about living in a world with limited eyesight. My hope is that family, friends and caregivers (professionals and non-professional) will share these 15 Vison Topics for Lifestyle Modifications. Together we can encourage the visually challenged to take advantage of attainable tools and technology in order to enrich their lives for a better future.

I also want to express loving gratitude to my daughter, Trina Marie Wyldeman, by acting as my technical liaison with Itty Bitty® Publishing, she made this book possible.

> "We are never really happy until we try to brighten the lives of others."
> ~ *Helen Keller*

Stop by our Itty Bitty® website to find
interesting blog entries regarding vision loss.

www.IttyBittyPublishing.com

Or contact Gloria Riley at

gloriariley321@gmail.com

What, I'm Losing My Sight?

Here are 15 essential things you need to know when losing your eyesight

Losing your eye sight as an adult is frightening. Your whole world is turned inside out and upside down. Everything you know about your physical surroundings is no longer real. It will impact you physically, mentally, and emotionally. There will also be an impact to your work life, your friendship structure and your family. In this Itty Bitty® book, Gloria Riley talks about the reality of sight loss, the changes it makes in your life and how to learn the skills you need going forward. She will help you set priorities to accept your immediate plight, and to always keep up hope.

After reading this book you will have:

- solutions to help fulfill specific needs,
- incentives to assist you in moving forward,
- beneficial resources that will shape your future.

If you or someone you know has lost, or is losing, their sight, pick up this Itty Bitty® book today and know that this is not the end of life, but the beginning of a new one!

Table of Contents

Introduction

Could YOU manage if you went blind in mid-life? It was estimated that 20 million Americans would lose vision because of macular degeneration, retinitis pigmentosa, and other age-related eye diseases by the end of 2020. That's 1 in every 15 people in the United States alone! According to the National Eye Institute, another 8 million Americans will be afflicted with vision impairments by the year 2050.

If your life has turned this corner, it will impact you physically, mentally, and emotionally. In this book, you will learn to express your feelings and frustrations to relieve associated stress. You must set your priorities to accept your immediate plight, but always keep up hope. Research and miracle cures are happening every day!

Modern technology has opened many windows for information on this subject. Yet sadly, many citizens remain uninformed of the various practical skills available to ease everyday-living challenges with vision loss.

In this Itty Bitty® Guidebook, you will find solutions to help fulfill specific needs, provide incentives, and provide beneficial resources that will help shape your future.

Note: <u>Baby Boomer Generation (1946 – 1964)</u>

Right now (2021), there are approximately 76 million Americans in this age range. As this population continues to age, more and more people will become susceptible to various degrees of diminishing eyesight and total blindness.

If you can't see the light, <u>become the light!</u>

Topic 1
Adjusting to Low Vision

Low Vision changes can be sudden or subtle. It can be a progressive disease, and your adjustments will become a work in progress should this happen to you. Once you have accepted the realization that you can't function in your usual ways any longer, you will have to make an honest assessment of your medical eye condition.

Setting goals and making plans are only the first steps toward success. You must be willing to follow through with hard work. Be willing to commit, listen and learn from your peers, and eye-service professionals. There are millions of folks who know what it is to walk in your shoes. Vision loss affects everyone, of all ages, from all walks of life, regardless of ethnicity, education, or financial status.

1. See an eye specialist as soon as you experience vision changes.
2. Learn all you can about your eye condition.
3. Ask your doctor: "How fast will my eye condition deteriorate?"
4. Many eye diseases can be prevented by regular annual eye checkups.

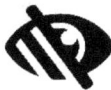

Tips: About "211"

"211" Information Centers are currently active in 50 states, the District of Columbia, Puerto Rico, and most of Canada. It is the most comprehensive source of information today. Referrals for every kind of need is also offered in 240 languages. Cut through the confusion by dialing "211" for private and public service agencies. Referral specialists will match the callers' needs with the available resources.

- Have an honest heart-to-heart conversation with yourself, your family, and your loved ones.
- If you're still employed, your employer is obligated by law, through the 1990 American Disabilities Act, to make reasonable accommodations in your work environment. This will prolong your career status.
- Ask what assistive aids and/or devices are available.
- Ask your doctor to refer you to local and state agencies that offer assistance for the visually impaired and the blind.

Topic 2
Simple Home Modifications

Before you get ahead of yourself you will need to review and reassess the familiar surroundings in your home. Surprisingly, the average person has no conception of the broad spectrum of sight. It's important to dispel the distorted belief of Blindness vs. Low Vision because most people believe that blindness implies a picture of total darkness. However, the levels of light, color, and imagery are unique to each individual. Clarity, color, and contrast may be affected separately or in combination. What you can see today may disappear into the shadows tomorrow. You will have to experiment until you find the proper adjustments that work for your personal needs.

1. Fluorescent lighting is the most commonly used light source in America. However, it contains a gas that causes flickering, which often results in health problems such as headaches, migraines, eye strain, stress, and anxiety.
2. In comparison, LED offers longevity, low cost, and low heat emission, which is a great safety feature. LED lighting is instantaneous making it increasingly popular.

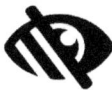

Tips: Balancing the Light and the Dark

- Gage the appearance of furnishings, décor, and carpets affected by the lighting changes throughout the day into night. Note the important features from top to bottom as familiar images may be swallowed by shadows.
- Be mindful of any sharp corners. Re-arrange furniture to avoid obstacles for a clearer walkway.
- Use curtains and blinds to control lighting glare.
- Brighten up those dark closets and countertops with stick-on lights.
- Illuminate indoor and outdoor walkways with motion sensor lighting.

Note: Remember, the best source of light is the Sun! Your body depends on sunlight to keep your bodies chemistry in balance. Without sun exposure many totally blind and visually impaired people are not able to sleep. This deficiency can result in a condition called "Non 24", which disrupts the body's circadian rhythm. Sleep deprivation then results in further negative health issues.

Topic 3
Organize Your Kitchen & Bathrooms

Consider clearing cluttered countertops in the kitchen and bathroom. Try using lightweight non-breakable dishware. By using a matched set, you can keep all your kitchen items uniform and stackable.

Do you have your own private bathroom, or do you share it? Avoid knocking things off the counters, by clearing all but essential items, such as a toothbrush. If you have a medicine cabinet, select one side of a shelf to place personal items. Then group hygiene products like mouth wash separately from medicines, such as aspirin.

1. Choose light color appliances for dark countertops.
2. Arrange light colored foods such as potatoes on a dark or colorful plate.
3. Try using color contrasting measuring cups, spoons, slicers, and peelers.
4. Replace kitchen rugs with endurance mats to eliminate slipping hazards.
5. Use nonslip bathroom mats and rugs.
6. Try a talking bathroom scale or a talking microwave!

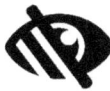

Tips: Keep Safety in Mind

- Pour liquids or measure dry goods on a tray for easier cleanup in case of spills.
- Avoid broken glass by using decorated metal tins or plastic storage containers.
- Replace drinking glasses with plastic cups or glassware.
- Tupperware® plastic products are still popular.
- Almost all grocery stores have plastic items available in the household section.
- Remember to duck! Be mindful of open kitchen cupboard doors.
- Close upright freezer doors and lowered dishwasher doors, too.
- Remember to use outreached hands if you're unable to distinguish any open doors.
- Be mindful of out-of-place tables and chairs.
- Remind family members to close all cabinet doors for your safety.

Topic 4
Household Hazards

Fall risks are the major household hazards for the visually impaired. Dangerous obstacles include area rugs and throw rugs. Catching your feet on a carpet edge may cause loss of balance, resulting in accidental falls.

Water splashed on floors, especially in the kitchen and on bathroom tile floors, can cause you to slip and fall. Many seniors, especially those who live alone, may not be able to call for help. You could find yourself lying on the floor for hours or even days before being discovered and rescued.

1. Install hand bars on bathtubs and handrails throughout living areas.
2. Handrails on outdoor stairways and walkways help keep you balanced.
3. Be mindful of indoor potted plants and trash cans placed in a room.
4. Remind children to pick up toys scattered on the inside and outside walk areas.
5. Consider wearing a waterproof medic alert. One press of a button will bring immediate "911" assistance right to your location, especially if you can't reach your phone.

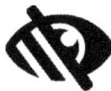

Tips: ABC's

- Avoid broken glass by using plastic or metal containers.
- Be mindful of small accessories sitting on the floors inside the house and outdoors.
- Consider removing throw rugs in the kitchen and bathrooms.

Topic 5
Labeling & Marking Systems

What do you do when your magnifying glass no longer helps you to read labels on canned goods? How many times have you put on an unmatched pair of socks? Try some old tricks and new techniques!

1. Finding a labeling and marking system that suits your needs can be something as simple as using buttons, rubber bands, or safety pins. They make excellent identifying markers. For example, you can distinguish a bottle of hair shampoo from a bottle of hair conditioner by using one band on the shampoo and two bands on the conditioner. Keep it simple!

2. There are products you can use on cloth, paper, plastic, metal, rubber, and wood surfaces. Great items are available to mark kitchen appliances. Some have raised marks that withstand heat from stovetops and are water-proof too.

3. Technology has evolved yesterday's tricks into amazing modern magic. Talking barcode readers and Smartphone apps snap photos of everyday items and speak the product name, description, and instructions. Amazing!

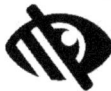

Tips: For Marking and Labeling

- Choose a labeling system that makes sense to you.
- Will pre-made labels convey enough information or will you need to create your own design?
- Choose from the diverse mixes of bump dots, glue dots, contrast tapes, and felt tapes.
- Velcro has two adhesive sides, one soft and the other wiry. It comes in circles, squares, and strips. Many products are available in variety packs.
- Safety pins can be attached discreetly under a shirt collar. Assign a pin size to determine the color. Assign one pin for white and two pins for blue shirts or tops.
- Button Magic attaches buttons on clothes without sewing. Choose a size and button shape to attach inside a pocket to designate a color code.
- Puff Paint comes in an easy applicator bottle. Simply apply a tactile dot on clothes. It dries fast and is waterproof. It can be found in craft stores and grocery stores.
- Try high-tech audio devices to improve and enhance your needs.
- Recruit someone sighted to help you label your items. Have fun together!

Topic 6
Personal Wardrobe

Sighted people take so many everyday routines
for granted, such as, grooming, dressing, and
maintaining a wardrobe. Vision impairment
should not become a barrier looking the way you
want to. Selecting a wardrobe is just as important
to men as it is to women.

Keeping your clothes organized for identification
purposes calls for a practical plan. Closets and
dresser drawers can be sectioned for speedy
recognition. Once you arrange your clothes
closet, you can make room for accessories.
Always return items to the same place every time.

1. Tell your personal assistant or caregiver
    your fashion style preference and color
    coordination likes and dislikes.
    Remember what it's like to see.
2. Whirlpool and Kenmore manufacture
    washer & dryers that have pitch tones in
    combination with easy to feel buttons and
    turn knobs. Another remarkable and
    inexpensive product is the Talking
    Laundry Module by General Electric.
    (GE®)

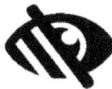

Tips: What's Your Hang Up?

- Classic wooden hangers are the most durable, while wire and plastic hangers will sag in time, causing clothes to stretch.
- Open-ended style hangers are best for pants and are sturdy enough to hold two pairs.
- Prevent wrinkles and creases in pants by using stainless steel hangers with rubber coating.
- Velvet lightweight suit hangers are perfect for women's tops or pants.
- Arrange clothes by season, color, formal, casual, mix & match.
- Pair matching pieces to make an outfit.
- Keep long sleeve shirts or blouses in the same closet zone.
- Use shoeboxes or plastic organizers for socks, ties, scarves, and gloves in dresser drawers.
- Safety pins keep matching socks together in drawers or for the laundry.
- Ice cube trays or egg cartons work great for organizing jewelry.

Topic 7
Getting Around – Mobility Aids

Low vision need not be confining. Tap into your GPS Mind Map as you venture out to mix and mingle in society. Electronic eyewear is accessible in today's marketplace. Two leading pioneers are: <u>esighteyewear.com and OrCam My Eye Pro.</u>

Sight, hearing and balance, each have a significant impact on mobility. Using a cane has several benefits as each style has a specific purpose. You will navigate differently outside well-known environments, but you are definitely capable!

1. Six cane styles include: a) White Canes, b) Red & White Striped Canes, c) Vibrational Canes, d) Symbol Canes, e) Guide Canes and f) Long Canes. These canes identify the carrier as blind or visually impaired. They are designed to detect obstacles, such as curbs, steps, posts, and trash bins.
2. Long Canes are customized for your height. By sweeping from side-to-side, the extra length alerts a warning for cracks in the pavements, cobblestones and other obstacles.

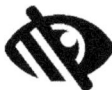

Tips: Grips and Cane Tips

- <u>Point tips</u>: Are used on canes to tap the ground around you searching for obstacles. This style is shaped like a piece of chalk, but it isn't as sensitive as the ball tip.
- <u>Ball tips</u>: Shaped like a small orange, the tip is moved from side-to-side with the ball rolling over the ground. It is sensitive to the conditions of the pavement.
- <u>Rollerball tips</u>: Glide well over surfaces and are smaller than the ball tip.
- <u>Folding support canes</u>: are adjustable for height and length allowing for better balance.
- <u>Grips:</u> are made from rubber, cork, or wood. Tips come in hook, threaded or slip-on.
- Quality canes are made from a variety of materials. Graphite rates number one followed by fiberglass, and aluminum.
- Consider a Guide Dog vs. a Human for a traveling companion.
- Implement the tactics you have just learned into your daily life and regain your self-confidence.

Topic 8
Recreation – Stay Active

The internet became the instant lifeline to keep us connected, while practicing social distancing during the 2020 global pandemic. Zoom groups formed to hold daily and weekly gatherings discussing important topics of concern. Already familiar with activity limitations, the blind community has embraced this new format.

1. Individual activities: Audio Books, Armchair Yoga, Armchair Travel Cruises, Podcasts, Radio Shows and Word Games. Outdoor activities include: Gardening, Golf, Swimming, and Hiking, or just plain Walking. Although some assistance may be required to navigate outdoors, these activities are very therapeutic. Consider becoming a Ham Radio Operator!

2. Group activities: Invite friends and family, or join a group, to play adaptive versions of many board and table games. Among them are Bingo, Card Games, Checkers, Dominoes Monopoly and Scrabble. If you're unable to attend a local Senior Center, enjoy your morning coffee with a group by Smartphone, iPad or using your computer.

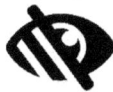

Tips: Elderhood Rocks!

- Use large print crossword magazines.
- Learn the 13 Braille letters used on Braille playing cards.
- Use a dark table or cloth for contrast when playing adaptive Dominoes. They are white with raised black dots.
- Some local and State Parks have specific hiking trails made for the visually impaired.
- Play Beep Ball – baseball adapted where all players are blindfolded whether they are totally blind or have partial vision. The ball and bases have sound sensors to alert the batter of the ball and base locations.
- Almost all local and State group communities for the blind, include people with low vision.
- VisionAware.org – offers recreational activities for seniors with vision challenges.
- AchillesInternational.org – provides volunteer coaches for bicycling, group walks, racing marathons, skiing, and sky diving. These are just some great avenues for staying healthy.

Topic 9
Caregivers – Family – Friends
How You Can Help

It's important to remember vision acuity, clarity, and sharpness differs with each individual. Some people only see through a fog or blur with one or both eyes. Some have no peripheral vision, while others only see through a center tunnel. Others have vision in part of an eye or one eye only. And some people have prosthetic eyes with literally no vision.

While some people are color blind, others can only see shapes and shadows, but no detail. Lighting, where there is no contrast, either very bright or very low, makes seeing details extremely difficult.

Etiquette awareness:

1. Have a hands-off attitude when you're going to try and help.
2. Introduce yourself first and then ask them if they need help.
3. Always ask someone first, if you might help to walk them across a street.
4. Never just grab them! You wouldn't grab someone who is sighted.

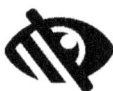

Tips: For How to Help

- Speak up! Let people know <u>how</u> you need them to help.
- People sometimes forget that low vision people can't do everything the same as the sighted.
- People with low vision live independent lives, but there are times they need assistance.
- When in an unfamiliar environment, a visually challenged person may need a few minutes to adjust before walking.
- It's important to be mindful that too much noise or commotion can be distracting. They will need extra time to concentrate and focus.

Topic 10
Accessibility Using Technology
Amazing Modern Adaptations

Online learning has taken a quantum leap. Huge potentials are being developed to enhance navigational skills and self-reliance.

1. Amazon Alexa – Introduced to the public in 2014 as an intelligent personal assistant, is capable of voice interaction.
2. EnhancedVision.com – carries low vision aids and electronic magnifiers that have helped thousands of people regain their visual independence. Search their website or call 1-800-811-3161.
3. GoodMaps – Designed specifically to navigate a large building or your home as an indoor GPS provides voice interaction and audible directions to your indoor destination. Download the GoodMaps Mobile App free of charge. Give it a try!
4. Northwest Access Fund – Provides low-interest loans for personal use, business, or equipment used in employment. Email: info@nwaccessfund.org Website: www.nwaccessfund.org or call 1-877-428-5116.

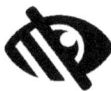

Tips: Your Moment of Choice

- Use Alexa (or Google Assistant) as a home automation system to control several smart devices.
- Choose the Compatible Plug Pack to turn lights on/off, set alarm reminders for the microwave, stove oven, coffee pot, heat controls, radio, and TV.
- Performance features include: Playing audiobooks, music, streaming podcasts, and making grocery lists. Alexa acts as a virtual assistant with AI technology. By simply calling her name she can provide current weather, traffic reports, sports, and other news information.
- Alexa can even sync your calendar to your smartphone.

Topic 11
Resources

There are several helpful resources available to you. Start with these informative links:

1. <u>IRPS</u> – Information Referral/Peer Support. Call Toll-free 1-800-424-8666 or Email: info@acb.org
2. <u>AccessablePharmacy</u>.com – Full-service home delivery specifically designed for the blind community. Pill packs available at no cost.
3. <u>Hadley School for the Blind</u> – Offers education and support free of charge. Call 1-800-323-4238 or Website: www.Hadley.edu
4. <u>Housing & Public Utilities Benefits</u> – The Federal Government Program website can connect you to energy assistance programs for your State. Website: www.benefits.gov
5. <u>National Library Service</u>: Offers access to books, magazines, and newspapers for those who are blind, visually impaired or whose physical limitations require use with Audio format. Call toll-free 1-888-657-7323 Website: www.loc.gov/nls/
6. <u>US Department of Veterans Affairs</u> – Services are free of charge. Call toll-free 1-844-698-2311. Website: www.va.gov

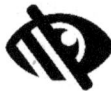

Tips: Catalogs & Online Shopping for low vision products

- Independent Living Aids – Call toll-free 1-800-537-2118.
- Maxi Aids Products – Download catalog (PDF) or request by mail. Call for information 1-631-752-0738 Website: www.maxiaids.com
- LS&S – For health care and mobility products. Call toll-free 1-800-468-4789 Website: www.LSSproducts.com
- BlindMiceMegaMall.com – Designated for screen readers and vision software. Call toll-free 1-866-922-8877
- TwoBlindBrothers.com: An online retail clothing website owned and operated by two visually impaired brothers.
- Enhanced Vision – Provides a diverse product line in the United States, United Kingdom, Germany, Japan, and Canada. Call 1-888-811-3161 Website: www.enhancedvision.com

Note: CANADA
- Canadian National Council of the Blind (CNIB) provides free programs to all Canadians. Call 1-800-265-4127 Website: www.cnib.ca
- Vision Loss Rehabilitation Canada - Call toll free 1-844-887-8572 Website: www.visionlossrehab.ca

Topic 12
Local, State, National & International Groups

Worldwide Social Media provides online educational courses, and expanding weekly events that are available at no cost to you.

1. <u>Local Groups</u>: Start by reaching out in your local community. No matter how large or small the population, groups are often affiliated with State and National Chapters. Check with your local libraries, churches, senior centers, and Lions Club.
2. <u>State Groups</u>: Expand your knowledge through leadership programs. Take advantage of educational programs and scholarships. Step up! Make a difference!
3. <u>National & International Groups</u>: <u>American Council for the Blind</u> Call toll-free 1-800-424-8666 Email: info@acb.org Website: www.acb.org <u>National Federation of the Blind</u>: Call 1-410-659-9314 Email: nfb@nfb.org Website: <u>www.nfb.org</u>
4. <u>Vision 2020: The Right to Sight</u>: is the global initiative for the elimination of avoidable blindness, a joint program of the World Health Organization (WHO).

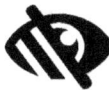

Tips: Hands Linked Together Around the Globe

- Each new day brings an opportunity for lifelong learning.
- Meet or make new friends at an online morning coffee social.
- Listen in on ACB Radio Mainstream.
- Expand your network and exchange ideas with friends.
- Sit in on group gatherings from coast-to-coast and around the world to share different interests and passions.
- Blind LGBT Pride International www.blindlgbtpride.org is an affiliate of American Council of the Blind. Reach out for support; we all matter!
- There are professional lounges for Attorneys and Teachers too.
- Technology Specialists offer information for low vision online learning.
- Blind Pen Pals International Facebook Group with 7.5K followers.

Topic 13
Fill in the Communication Gap

It's a fact that large cities afford more opportunities, but what about those who live in rural communities and live more sheltered lives? If there are no self-help support groups in your area, seriously consider starting one.

1. Select a safe and comfortable meeting place to encourage folks to express themselves.
2. Before opening the meeting, establish the intentions of the group and provide rules of etiquette. Ensure an atmosphere of safety and that a sense of welcome is extended to all your group participants.
3. Keep an open-minded attitude of the group as a whole. Listen and be respectful of others' shared experiences. We all have a story and it is important to acknowledge our common visual challenges.
4. Remain sensitive to introverted and shy individuals. The intent to share your stories, frustrations, and successes bring many blessings to all who are willing to persevere in the continued struggle of adjusting to vision loss.

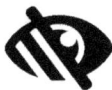

Tips: Get the word out

- Use local newspaper monthly calendar of events.
- Place flyers in the library, local eye/medical offices, and hospital bulletin boards.
- Utilize grocery store and post office bulletin boards.
- Place announcements in Sunday Church bulletins.
- Assist newcomers by describing the room layout. Have each participant introduce themselves and give a short explanation of why they came to the meeting.
- Let first-timers know they are welcome to listen only if they are not comfortable sharing.
- Become a good listener.
- Show interest in each individual.
- Avoid jumping to conclusions.
- Develop trust by sharing your personal experiences.
- Be tolerant and sensitive to the fears, frustrations and visual challenges of others.
- Offer to remain after the meeting to help with clean-up.

Topic 14
Building Firm Foundations
Support Groups vs. Professional Counseling

When shattering events bring changes into your personal life, you are changed emotionally, physically, and spiritually and are no longer the same. You can find yourself at a fork in your life path. As you forge into uncharted territory, you will choose your direction. However, you alone have to walk it. You will find yourself torn between two worlds. You may have never been exposed to the blind community and the thought is frightening. Common feelings of anger, denial, and depression can surface. There is assurance and comfort when talking with people who understand what you are going through.

1. A peer support group for low vision is a great place to ask questions about blind culture and exchange information.
2. Not everyone feels comfortable in a peer group setting. Professional Counseling is another option where you can have guaranteed confidentiality. Persons who are certified and licensed to practice in these professions must follow the specific code of ethics. Insurance and payment options are generally available.

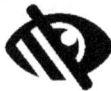

Tips: Advice & Encouragement

- Search deep to find your inner strength.
- Rise to the challenge and try new ideas.
- Stay grounded and focused.
- Build meaningful connections.
- Become a new version of yourself.
- Claim your new destiny.
- Retain your self-identity.
- Keep a sense of humor.
- Peer groups are not facilitated by a health care professional.

Topic 15
Reach Out to Advocate

If you have experienced the benefits of a self-help group, speak out to be heard, be seen, inform, and educate the public to establish a positive image of persons who are legally blind and visually impaired.

1. Take the first step and join a local group chapter or affiliate for your State. These are all educational experiences, adding to knowledge and skills that will enhance your leadership opportunities.
2. Choose a committee and get involved in your community.
3. Express your interest to the nominating committee that you are interested in running for office. You can lead your group by setting goals and intentions. Share your vision to further the cause for optical challenges. Shine a light on the path shadowed by darkness for those who struggle now and those who will stumble in the future. You will follow some big footsteps, but you can make big imprints of your own!

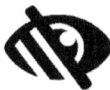

Tips: Start Something Priceless!

- By sharing tips, techniques, and technology you can live a more productive and independent life.
- Provide a forum for discussions.
- Partner with your City to promote informed decisions of community issues by airing monthly programs on local talk shows and the City's website.
- Analyze community issues for the needs of your group.
- How many busy street corners have talking crosswalk signals?
- Leadoff a project survey and report your needs to your City Council.
- Promote Recognition Days.
- National Guide Dog Month – September.
- White Cane Day – October 15th annually Observes precautions for drivers of motor vehicles, wheelchair users for pedestrians who are using a white cane or service animal. (Some Lions Clubs celebrate this during the month of May).
- World Sight Day – 2nd Thursday of October annually. Focus is global attention on visual impairment/blindness. Celebrates achievements and advocates for increased attention to eye care globally.

You've finished. Before you go…

Tweet/share that you finished this book.

Please star rate this book.

Reviews are solid gold to writers. Please take a few minutes to give us some itty bitty feedback.

ABOUT THE AUTHOR

Gloria Riley was born with an incurable, hereditary eye disease. At age 16, her older brother took her to an eye specialist. Dr. Fortier confirmed the same diagnosis that her brother had lived with for 30 years. As the result of this exam, Gloria finally received a proper pair of prescription eyeglasses. For the first time in her life, she was able to clearly distinguish the individual leaves growing on trees. Before then, tree leaves were only seen as a green blur!

Even with glasses, Gloria has never experienced 20/20 vision. Every eye appointment was a challenge because her vision was literally off the charts! Today, her remaining vision with glasses is only 10%.

She retired from a distinguished career as a "911" Communications Officer and Supervisor, working in California and Oregon. After the passing of her husband, she relocated to Bellingham, Washington to be near her only daughter. It was there that she discovered the best-kept secret in town, the United Blind of Whatcom County. (UBWC)

A whole new world opened for her through the incredible people in this small non-profit organization. Once she got involved and by sharing experiences, soon discovered how many different ways other people, just like her, learned to manage their daily lives with hope, happiness, and humor.   Not only was she elected President of UBWC in 2014, but she also became a "Newsline" editor for the affiliate, Washington Council of the Blind in 2015. During the same year, she was asked to facilitate the Visually Impaired Persons (VIP) support group at the Gipson Senior Center in Everett, Washington.

You are welcome to share coffee and conversation at the Shadow Light Café, Gloria's Facebook Group or
Email: gloriariley321@gmail.com

If you enjoyed this Itty Bitty® book you might also like…

- **Your Amazing Itty Bitty® What Happens When Book** – Sharón Lynn Wyeth

- **Your Amazing Itty Bitty® Fear-Busting Book** – Lucetta Zayton

- **Your Amazing Itty Bitty® Health and Wellness Experts Book** – Various Authors

And Coming Soon!
Your Amazing Itty Bitty® Losing Your Vision Book – Katie Friedman, LOD

Or any of the other Amazing Itty Bitty® books available on line at www.ittybittypublishing.com